How to Live for 100 Years With

The right Diet

Prevent Chronic Illness and Live Well by

Eating the Right Food

TABLE OF CONTENT

INTRODUCTION

Modern man has drifted far away from nature. He leads a hectic life full of tension, eats junk food, drinks polluted water and indulges in all sorts of excesses. No wonder ill-health is on the rise. Diseases come as a natural punishment. The number and varieties of items of eatables and drinks are multiplying day by day. Moreover, we become gluttonous at late night parties. Today's life is a life of hast, hurry, bustle and mental tension. Consequently the mode of men's life has become regular and discordant. Biological rhythm of the body is endangered by irregular timings of eating, drinking, sleeping and walking. These irregularities disarrange the excretory functioning of the body, leading to common complaints of constipation, insomnia, body ache and headache. Intoxicating substances like tea and coffee accumulates toxins and other harmful elements in the body. The system of adding color, taste and flavor to food and the various processes through which it passes destroy its life-giving nutrients. Synthetic vitamins are added to make it nutritious. But all these additives and processed foods are injurious to health. To get rid of diseases man resort to poisonous drugs and deadly chemicals which ultimately disable or kill him.

Thus, in trying to escape diseases man becomes a victim of drugs and medicines. He can save himself if only he knows the fact that right food has exceptionally healing properties. Natural food can be used effectively to prevent as well as cure diseases. Healing powers of fresh fruit and vegetable juices can't be denied. This is because they contain a huge amount of nourishing and disease fighting nutrients like: Vitamins, Minerals and Enzymes.

So correctly stated by the Father of Medicine, the famous Greek Physician, Hippocrates, " Let thy food be thy medicine." Socrates too stated "Diet is health, Diet is medicine." We all wish to live a healthy, happy life free from all diseases, but very few of us make right and serious effort in this direction. Nature has provided a variety of food items to us, but instead of making them part of our diet, we prefer hot and spicy food, which is dangerous to the health of mankind. Juice diet, especially, can cure us of chronic diseases and keep our mind and body healthy. Naturopathy or Nature-cure has been gaining increasing popularity during the last few years, and particularly, juice therapy has its exclusive importance in Nature cure. Where medicines and injections fail to cure a disease, a proper diet, vegetables and fruit juices show miraculous results.

A consideration of what we eat and why we eat it has becoming more urgent and important than it has ever been in the history of modern lifestyle. The food and physical activity choices individuals make on a daily basis affects their health. This effect is about today, tomorrow and in the future. This is no brainier as countless studies have shown that most critical diseases that affects humans today are linked to what these humans put through their mouth. This speaks of hypertension, cardiovascular disease, diabetes and such other ailments. This without doubt means dietary guidelines are more than ever needed in our society today.

A lot of people eat plenty of foods yet sadly this plenty of food is not the right type of food. These foods do not give the body the nutrients needed to be healthy. Take for instance the excessive eating of sugar. Sugar is harmful in excess and has been shown to even cause weight gain. Yet a lot of people eat a lot of sugar without restraint in sodas they drink, cakes they eat and so on. The secret to weight gain is that whatever the body can not expend will be added as extra weight. Activity is what will burn any extra calories that we eat. This will be less necessary should we eat the right foods in the first place.

The attitude today amongst a lot of people especially the younger ones is that eating right and being physically active are just a diet and physical program. On the contrary they are actually keys to a healthy lifestyle. This healthy lifestyle will drastically reduce the risk of chronic diseases that are reaching epidemic levels in most parts of the world such as heart disease, diabetes,osteoporosis, cancers and hypertension. Ensuring that you stay within the daily calorie limit the most suitable way and recommended by experts to giving your body a balanced nutrition it requires is when you eat a variety of nutrient rich foods on a daily basis. What makes up a healthy eating plan is known and apparent;

a. Be biased towards abundant fruits, veggies, whole grains, and fat-free or low-fat milk and milk products.

b. Include lean meats, poultry, fish, beans, eggs and nuts in your meals.

c. Eat a diet low in cholesterol, trans facts, saturated fats, sodium (found in many salts) and added sugars.

Watch what you eat. Eating the right things in the right portions can potentially give you an expanded life on this earth. You will be much healthier. Heart disease can be a non factor if you eat right. Diabetes can be controlled if you eat what you are supposed to. Keeping your weight where it should be will by getting the right nutrition can do wonders for your blood pressure. No matter how old or young you are, eating right can be started at any time in your life. It is just a matter of how bad you are when you decide to start getting the sustenance you should be putting into your body.

Stay active. Staying physically active can go a long way in the prevention of up to 6 things.

Things like depression, osteoporosis and depression. Walking, running, they do the same thing.

You have to walk fast. You have to do it for a half hour without any breaks. You may want to take up bike riding. You may want to swim. Get out there and be active.

Eating right and staying active could keep you alive until the ripe old age of 90 or longer. Just do not over do it. Getting an injury will set you back. Start out slowly and work your way up to more aggressive things.

How to Live for 100 Years With The right Diet

Prevent Chronic Illness and Live Well by Eating the Right Food

CHAPTER ONE
WHAT ARE CHRONIC DISEASE AND CAUSES

Chronic Disease is a slow progressive disease with a long duration that comes in a variety of forms such as: Heart Disease, Stroke, Cancer, Respiratory Disease, Obesity, and Diabetes. Chronic Disease is the No. 1 Killer of Humans worldwide annually. It affects millions of people worldwide. Research and technology exists to end the disease, but humans lack the resources and the will to make healthy lifestyles choices. You could say that Chronic Disease is a mental and emotional disease with physical consequences.

Chronic Disease is seen as a social ill where the major risk factors are: unhealthy diet, physical inactivity, alcoholism, anxiety, depression, stress, or tobacco use. The global medical scientific community doesn't see Habitual Disease as being infectious or a pandemic, so no resources are being used to eliminate or resolve them.

Yet, both of them pose a far greater problem for humanity and medical science than do any infectious diseases. If the major risk factors for persistent disease were eliminated, at least 80% of heart disease, stroke and type two diabetes would be prevented; and 40% of all cancers would be eliminated.

Humans and animals experience sickness/illness as the body's attempt to get our attention that there is an imbalance. We experience a condition, symptom or feeling, e.g., runny nose, headache, fatigue, back pain. Signs are always present, but we are not trained how to see or identify them. We only recognize them when they are tied to a big red flag or the body or an organ stops functioning.

Many ailments have an onset of twenty to thirty years before showing any outward signs, e.g., cancer, fibromyalgia, heart attack, stroke. YES! The absence of symptoms or physical signs does not equate to being healthy.

How do you acquire Chronic Disease?

The disease occurs when people lack adequate treatment and education about the effects of social ills that all too frequently accompany economic and urban development, e.g., effects of tobacco, cancer, pollution, stress, eating problems, depression, alcohol, drug use, suicide, violence, anger, and mental and emotional pain. The disease does not spread from person to person, but leaves the burden with each individual dependent on their abilities to seek treatment or support.

How is Chronic Disease treated?

The World Health Organization (WHO), nations, governments, communities, and organizations in the private and public sectors have been trying to get the upper hand with Chronic Disease for over 80 years. The disease claims more than 40 Million lives annually and half of the deaths are
under 70 years old and female. By far, Chronic Disease is the leading cause of mortality worldwide, representing over 60% of all deaths annually and rising.

There are two schools of thought:

Complementary & Alternative Medicine sees Chronic Disease as an energy imbalance within the body that affects all areas of the body: physical, emotional, mental, and spiritual. A holistic treatment plan considers an integrative approach to: identify the causes of the energy imbalances, provide individualized remedies and therapies, prevent recurrence, and reintegrate health and wellness.

This is accomplished through the use of Integrative Medicine, which is the collaboration of Energy, Complementary/Alternative, and Allopathic Medicines. The solution to any imbalance within the body is seen as a process and not a destination. The alleviation of all physical symptoms doesn't mean that the imbalance is resolved.

Allopathic (Western) Medicine American Medical Association (AMA), American Psychiatric Association (APA), and Pharmaceutical Research & Manufactures of America (Big Pharma) have labeled the symptoms and effects of Chronic Disease as a Disorder or Syndrome. The APA's Diagnostic & Statistical Manual of Mental Disorders (DSM) refers to Chronic Disease as physical dysfunction or mental disorder. Once labeled then the use of drugs, invasive surgery, or clinical therapy can be applied to treat the symptoms and effects of the habitual disease. Meanwhile, the causes of the persistent disease and imbalances within the body are never addressed.

What are some other forms of Chronic Disease?

The WHO has stated that Chronic Disease needs to be seen in the same light as an infectious pandemic, in order for the international scientific community to take action and acquire the necessary funding. The WHO has indicated that this is not a complete list. It is only the tip of the iceberg for chronic (mental, emotional, physical) diseases:

Addictions

Alzheimer's

Arthritis

Autoimmune Diseases

Cancer (all forms)

Cardiovascular Disease

Chronic Fatigue

Combat Stress

Cystic Fibrosis

Diabetes

Eating Disorders (overeating, anorexia, bulimia, Obesity)

Epilepsy & Seizures

Fibromyalgia

Heart Disease, Stroke

Hypertension, Stress,

Influenza & Pneumonia

Kidney Disease

Osteoporosis

Parkinson's

Post Traumatic Stress

Pulmonary Disease

Respiratory Disease

Sexual Assault, Rape

Suicide

Chronic Disease crosses all education, social economic, cultural, rural, and urban barriers. It infects and erodes personal lives, the lives of families, and devastates communities as well as nations. Since Chronic Disease is not considered a pandemic or infectious disease it does not attract the medical science community at a local or global level.

Prevention of Chronic Diseases With Diet and Nutrition

In a recently published study conducted by the acclaimed WHO Study Group of Canada, the results continually pointed back to the importance of diet and nutrition in the fight against ongoing and chronic diseases. After a year of testing and research including a control group and a placebo-mandated group, the association found that there are direct and irrevocable links between dieting, nutrition, and chronic diseases.

Hope Through Healthier Lifestyles

The prevention of diseases that is persistent and popular with the citizens of the United States as well as Canada, show that through a healthy lifestyle there is hope. There is a combined positive affect from those that watch what they eat and the downward cycle of diseases such as myocardial infarction and stomach ulcers.

Diet Factor

The study recognized and labeled at least a dozen core reasons for individuals that suffer one or more form of the chronic diseases listed above. The diet factor as long as this regiment was linked with a proper nutritional backing showed massive improvements across the board for those that looked after their bodies.

Dietary and lifestyle choices are very bad in the United States with Canada fairing slightly healthier on aspects such as nutrition derived from fruits and vegetables. When combined with a regular exercise program it demonstrated a spike in health and a lowering of cases of chronic disease.

The prevention of chronic diseases through dieting and nutrition has grabbed many research institution's attention throughout not only North America but also the world. As food sources and sustenance farming practices improve so goes the health and nutritional intake of a greener, leaner planet.

It has been shown that during the past decade, from 2000-2010, the number of people suffering from obesity and heart disease has climbed higher but slower than the previous decade.

The conclusion of this study by WHO demands that if people who considering themselves likely candidates for genetically predisposed heart conditions and other chronic diseases, would eat healthier that the rates would drop even lower throughout the next decade. The importance of eating nutritiously has always been a fact and not surprising when a research study demonstrates the connectiveness of diet and nutrition to chronic diseases. The prevention of chronic diseases through better eating and healthier lifestyle habits will be center stage.

Chronic Disease Management

Many people seek to learn more about chronic disease management. This is especially true regarding those currently suffering from a medical condition or those that are at a high risk of getting one. Dietary supplements are typically aids that help you to get the right nutrients you need each day. Some people use them often when they cannot eat a certain type of food, or at least do not eat enough of it to get the recommended daily allowance.

Supplements typically come in a pill form, but can also be administered in a powder or liquid. The most common supplements that people take along with their diet include those for vitamins, protein, and fiber. These can be taken when the person is not receiving enough of the nutrients from the food he/she consumes.

Supplements have been found to aid in chronic disease management. This is because they provide your body with the nutrients that it needs to stay healthy. Fish oil, for example, is a common supplement that provides the body with fatty acids. Good sources of fat keep you healthy by reducing bad cholesterol as well as promoting an increase in the good cholesterol. This can help prevent hardening of the arteries that could lead to a heart attack or cardiovascular disease.

Studies have been conducted to test a number of different supplements to find the benefits of including them in your diet. Many have been found to help reduce the chances of you getting a chronic disease in one way or the another. Supplements, like the fish oil mentioned above, work to keep your body healthy. This assistance can help to reduce your risk of contracting a serious medical condition. Other things that supplements can help you avoid include high blood pressure, stroke, kidney failure, and heart disease.

It is important to note that you still need to maintain a well balanced diet, even if you do use supplements for chronic disease management. The best source of vitamins and minerals are the foods we consume at each meal. The supplements will help to fill in the gaps as far as the important nutrients our bodies need. However, it is always best to shoot for getting most of the substances from food rather than a dietary aid.

As you can see, supplements can help keep you from developing a chronic disease.

They can also assist in controlling any serious condition you have. They have been known to help keep the body healthy so that your risk of getting a disease is lowered. It is essential that you only use the supplements as an assisting tool, and not your sole method for acquiring certain minerals, unless you cannot eat the foods that will give you the nutrients in a natural manner.

Prevent and Control Chronic Disease Through Lifestyle Interventions

Scientific evidence suggests the importance of adhering to a disciplined lifestyle approach to prevent and control chronic disease. Faulty and imbalanced diets and eating habits, lack of physical activity and smoking are confirmed risks for chronic diseases. Obesity, hypertension and high cholesterol levels have certain biological risks which have been confirmed as risk factors for heart disease, diabetes and stroke. Significant biological risk factors can continue to affect the health and quality of life of the next generation Physical activity and nutrient consumption throughout life influence genes and may define susceptibility to illness and disease. The global health trend has been in the increase in risk factors which affect obesity, physical activity.

Some preventive steps taken in early life offer lifelong health benefits. Preventive lifestyle interventions are more effective if they extend beyond individual risk factors and continue throughout the course of life. Improvement in eating patterns, diets and physical exercise in adults and senior citizens will reduce the risk of chronic diseases from death and disability.

A complementary secondary strategy to use diet and physical activity to retard existing chronic disease from progressing and reducing death rate and disease burden. Pay attention to and address the risk factors for chronic diseases throughout your lifespan. Primary prevention interventions aim to shift the profile of the whole population in a healthier direction. Small changes made to reduce risk factors in a majority of people who are at moderate risk can have a huge impact on their life quality and well being. According to the World Health Organisation, improved lifestyles reduce the risk for diabetes by a striking 58% over 4 years. Studies have shown that up to 80% of heart disease cases and 90% type 2 diabetes cases could be avoided through positive lifestyle interventions. One-third of cancers can be avoided if you eat health, maintain normal weight and exercise regularly. So, get started by eating right and get moving with a regular exercise plan to stay healthy lifelong.

Is Chronic Disease Is Preventable?

The WHO considers the top 5 causes of death to all be chronic disease-all of which are preventable, or at least delay-able. And they are not the only ones. The US centers for Disease Control and Prevention (CDC) and most major health authorities world-wide agree. To fight the ever increasing risk and presence of chronic disease we need to do three things: Stop Smoking, Get Active, and FIX OUR DIETS!!!!!!!

Top Five Causes of Death World Wide Are All "Chronic Diseases"

Heart Disease

Cancer

Stroke

Chronic respiratory disease

Diabetes

The WHO sees nutrition as the foundation of health. The formula is simple and compelling poor nutrition equals poor health and greater disease. Good nutrition equals good health and less disease. It's simple and it's irrefutable.

Fruits, Vegetables, Grains And Fish Hold The Keys To Prevention.

Healthy whole foods and the powerful protector nutrients they contain are the arsenal the WHO, the CDC, THE USFDA, the American Heart Association, the U.S. National Cancer Institute, and others point to as our best weapons in the fight against chronic disease.

For heart Disease and Stroke prevention the American Heart Association recommends: **Vegetables and fruits**: eating a variety of fruits and vegetables may help you control your weight and your blood pressure.

Whole grain foods: contains fibre that can help lower your blood cholesterol and help you feel full, which may help you manage your weight.

Fish: at least twice a week. Recent research shows that eating oily fish containing omega-3 fatty acids (for example, Salmon, trout, and herring) may help lower your risk of death from coronary artery disease.

For cancer prevention the U.S. National Cancer Institute says:

- Populations with diets high in fruits and vegetables tend to have a lower cancer risk.

- Fruits, vegetables and grains contain a number of nutrients, including carotenoids, vitamin-A, and vitamin-c.

- Numerous studies have found evidence that carotenoids reduce the risk of some cancers.

For Diabetes prevention the American Diabetes Association recommends:

Eat lots of vegetables and fruits. Try picking from the rainbow of colours available to maximize variety. Eat non starchy vegetables such as spinach, carrots, broccoli or green beans with meals.

A long life is a life well spent

CHAPTER TWO
CONTRACTING DIABETES

Many people, especially those whose families the disease runs in, want to know how they can prevent diabetes. Knowing and understanding exactly what causes diabetes is the first step in preventing the disease from taking hold. The causes of this disease really have more to do with the way that you live your life than with any hereditary factors.

What this means is that how can you prevent diabetes is primarily through eating right, and avoiding a sedentary lifestyle. It has been proven that up to 90% of the people that develop Type II diabetes are overweight, and that maintaining a healthy weight balance can be one of the most powerful deterrents of this disease. Even if your weight does stay within a moderate range you can still fall victim to this disease. Primarily, what causes diabetes Type II is many years of abusing your digestive system through a high intake of junk foods, fats, and preservatives.

This usually leads to obesity, but not in every case. Some people are able to maintain a reasonable bodyweight due to possessing a high metabolism, but it is due to the body not receiving the nutrients that it needs.

How can you prevent diabetes?

Diabetes Type II is first and foremost a nutritional disease, and that means that in order to prevent this ailment from taking control of your life you have to make sure that you are taking in all of the vitamins and minerals that your body requires, together with the proteins, carbohydrates, and other essential nutrients that your body needs in order to be healthy.

Since we know that what causes diabetes is a diet lacking in essential nutrients what can we do? Eating better is the main thing, but supplementing your diet with all natural health supplement that is designed specifically towards giving you the nutrients that are necessary in order to ward the disease off, or alleviate your complications from the disease if you have already been diagnosed is of the utmost importance also.

How can you prevent diabetes? Through the use of supplements that are formulated to make your insulin production and secretion is more efficient, regenerate insulin producing cells in the pancreas, produce more efficient blood sugar uptake, and reduce the risk of potentially fatal diabetes related diseases is the answer. These types of products can truly make a difference in your life, and you should take advantage of the power that they possess.

What many people do not realize is you can avoid, or at least manage, diabetes with what you consume. Now, this is not to say that Type-1 diabetes can be controlled in the same manner. There is a great difference between diabetes that is genetic and Type-2 diabetes that is caused by a poor diet and unhealthy weight gain.

Your body needs glucose for energy. When you have Type-2 diabetes, this glucose builds up in the blood stream rather than being reasonably distributed, by insulin, to the cells throughout the body. When you consume too much sugar and gain too much weight, your body "forgets" how to produce the insulin needed to perform this function. Without this insulin, the sugars you eat build up in the blood stream causing even further complications.

Type-2 diabetes is a little more complicated than this, but this is the basic process. So, as you can see, it can be quite dangerous and very scary. Since this process can be controlled, monitored, and maintained, it is worth taking the steps to try to avoid this life altering disease. One of the greatest things you can do for yourself is to start working out. Exercise is the absolute best medicine for many different ailments throughout the body; and will help to prevent many negative side effects of aging.

The next thing you need to do is watch what you eat. First things first, you should be consuming between 1800 and 2000 calories a day. Even if you are trying to lose weight you should never cut calories less than 1500 calories. Finding the right caloric intake for your body may take a few weeks; just make sure you do not overdo it.

Secondly, you need to start eating the right kind of foods; foods known as clean foods. Foods that can be found in nature like fruits, vegetables, meats, dairy products, and nuts and grains are exactly what you should be filling your body with. It is time to say goodbye to restaurant foods fast and processed foods; you know, the ones that line the most of the shelves in any supermarket.

On top of this you should make sure that you eat 5-6 times a day, or every few hours. See, eating in this manner will naturally help balance out your blood sugar levels. It also keeps your body functioning at optimal levels allowing it to continue to produce the hormones you need, which includes insulin production and performance.

So, whether you are worried about diabetes or not, you should be. This disease can kill you and will change your life. Rather than try to change your life after you contract the disease, change your life now. Make the right lifestyle choices, start eating right, and watch yourself become healthier as they days go by.

Types Of Diabetes And The Causes Of Diabetes

Diabetes is considered a silent killer if left unnoticed or untreated. The symptoms are exhibited only after the patient develops health related issues. Diabetes is a condition where excess glucose is produced in the body.

The pancreas is unable to produce enough insulin or the hormone producing insulin to control sugar levels in the body. The excess sugar produced within the blood is therefore not under control. As the insulin level decreases, the sugar level in the body increases. This causes long term damages to many parts of the body and may even lead to death. There are many different types and causes of diabetes.

Glucose is an important constituent for the proper functioning of the body as it produces the required energy for routine activities such as working, exercising and other day to day chores. However, if glucose is produced in excess and it is not regulated by insulin it causes harm to the body. Glucose is obtained from the food intake and released into the blood by the liver. Insulin produced by the pancreas in a healthy person is usually sufficient to regulate the sugar levels. In a diabetic, the insulin is not enough or the usage is improper.

There are many types and causes of Diabetes:

Type-1 Diabetes: In this condition, the pancreas secretes very little insulin or completely stops producing insulin as the cells that control the sugar levels in the body are dead. This occurs as the body attacks and kills its own cells in the pancreas and this condition is known as the autoimmune reaction. Type 1 diabetes is caused due to many factors including alcohol consumption, infection or disease, removal of the pancreas by surgery and so on. This diabetes type can occur in children due to genetic reasons and in juveniles due to stress or hereditary reasons. Those affected with type 1 Diabetes are required to take daily insulin to survive.

Type-2 Diabetes: In this condition the pancreas produce insulin but the cells receiving the insulin fail to be stimulated and this results in insulin resistance. As a result, there is an increase in the production of insulin and this may result in insufficient levels of insulin to control sugar level in the body. Type 2 diabetes generally affects adults. The causes of diabetes of this type include aging, being over weight and physical inactivity.

This type of diabetes need not depend on insulin treatment but with proper diet, exercise and oral medication, it can be kept under long-term control.

Gestational Diabetes: This type of diabetes usually occurs during pregnancy and ends after the birth of the child. A woman who suffers from gestational diabetes has a lot of insulin in the body. However, certain hormones produced during gestation blocks the usage of insulin thereby creating an imbalance in sugar level.

Juvenile Diabetes: Juvenile diabetes is when the pancreas produces little or no insulin in a child.

The causes of diabetes in juveniles are generally hereditary.

How Can You Prevents Diabetes?

Dealing with diabetes can be frustrating, so it's in your best interest to learn how you can prevent this disease. Today there is no cure for this problem yet, so taking some steps to prevent it can be important, especially since it is the sixth top cause of death in the U.S. today.

Some people deal with more risk factors than others for diabetes, but no matter your risk factors, there are some simple steps you can take to help prevent dealing with diabetes.

Keep Your Weight Down: First of all, one of the most important things that you can do is to make sure you keep your weight down at a healthy level. Many people today who end up dealing with diabetes are overweight, which is a huge problem. When you are too heavy, your risk of dealing with diabetes can be drastically increased. So, work on keeping your weight at a level that is healthy for you.

Exercise Regularly: Exercising on a regular basis is also important if you want to prevent dealing with diabetes. When you exercise on a regular basis, it helps to keep your weight down and can keep your blood flowing as you should. If you have family members who already have diabetes, then exercising regularly is especially important for you.

Eat Right: Eating right is another thing that you can do to prevent diabetes as well. Your diet should be one that is low in sugar and fat. You should restrict the amounts of starches and glucose that you take in as well, since diabetes includes problems with the body producing or using insulin.

Have a Checkup Regularly: Having a checkup regularly is important as well, since doctors can help let you know whether you have risk factors for diabetes or if you are a borderline diabetic. You should have your blood glucose measured every couple of years, especially after you get over the age of 45. This is especially important if you have a family history or diabetes or you are already overweight.

Eat More Fruits and Veggies: Eating more fruits and vegetables can also help you to prevent diabetes as well. There are studies out there that actually show that the pigments that give veggies their color can help to stimulate the production of insulin in the body.

Keep Blood Pressure Down: Keeping your blood pressure down is imperative if you want to prevent diabetes. Many people who have high blood pressure end up with diabetes, and if you have high blood pressure, you should work on lowering it so you can avoid dealing with diabetes.

Diabetes is a problem that is serious and that you'll definitely want to work to prevent. While you may have some of the risk factors already, you can work to prevent this from happening to you. When you eat right, exercise, keep your weight down, and have regular checkups, you can better prevent dealing with diabetes. So make sure that you follow these simple steps to help prevent diabetes in your life.

CHAPTER THREE
HIGH CHOLESTEROL LEVELS

Many people today wonder what are the causes of high cholesterol, and what the high cholesterol symptoms are. These are good questions to ask, as levels above normal can lead to high blood pressure, clogged arteries, and ultimately strokes and heart disease, the leading killers of Americans today.

Unfortunately, cholesterol levels above normal does not have symptoms as we normally think of them (headaches, shortness of breath, etc). It is possible for dangerously high cholesterol to be completely silent and undetectable, and for people to only find out their levels are too high when and if they are tested for it. Even worse, when you do develop "symptoms" (as we normally think of them), it's a big danger sign. At this point, you would be feeling symptoms of other health problems, like an oncoming heart attack or stroke, rather than high cholesterol symptoms themselves.

Lifestyle causes

There are, however, some lifestyle choices that lead to bad cholesterol levels. If you meet more than half of the risk factors below, you might want to have your cholesterol levels tested during your next medical check-up.

Lifestyle causes of high cholesterol include:

Your family has a history of heart problems

You eat fatty meals (fat food, whole milk, cheese, bacon, etc.)

You are overweight (your body stores more fat and cholesterol than it burns)

You get little exercise

You smoke

You drink more than two alcoholic beverages a day

The good thing about lifestyle choices like diet, exercise, weight, and smoking leading to cholesterol problems is that they are reversible. You can reduce your risk of developing high levels (or, if you already have bad cholesterol, lower your levels) by changing your lifestyle. Eating a low-fat diet, getting daily cardiovascular exercise (even just walking), losing weight, and quitting smoking can all reduce those levels.

Biological Causes

Unfortunately, there are other causes of high cholesterol that we can do little about. These risk factors are biological or genetic. Although you can do little to change them, being aware of these risk factors is the closest you can come to recognizing high cholesterol symptoms.

The biological causes of high cholesterol include:

Illnesses: There are a few medical conditions that lead to this type of problem, such as an under active thyroid, or kidney and liver diseases. These, however, can quickly be tested and either confirmed or ruled out by your doctor.

Heredity: Some families are genetically prone to increased blood lipid levels. If there is a history of heart disease in your family history, you may be prone to it too.

If your readings are high, look for natural ways to lower it. The vast majority of cases of high cholesterol can be lowered by taking the right supplements and making changes in the diet. Medication should be used only when all else fails.

Age: As both women and men grow older, their levels slowly rise. Around ages 60 to 65, cholesterol levels level off and stop increasing. In other words, the older you are, the greater your chance of having high cholesterol level.

Gender: Women generally have lower cholesterol levels than men of the same age. After they reach menopause, usually around age 50, women generally have higher cholesterol levels than men of the same age.

Stress: Medical studies have found that long-term stress can raise cholesterol levels. This may be due, however, to how people handle stress-for example, smoking or comfort eating of fatty foods may be the causes of high cholesterol, not the stress itself.

Finally, remember this: since high cholesterol symptoms are silent and unnoticeable, the best way to avoid more serious conditions like heart disease or strokes is simply to check your cholesterol levels regularly, and avoid the causes of high cholesterol that lead to developing high cholesterol symptoms in the first place.

Eventually almost everyone will experience the problem of having high cholesterol but having high cholesterol as a result of a bad diet is simply inexcusable. For most of us it is nearly impossible to eat a totally healthy diet all of our lives since we don't have the resolve of Jack LaLanne who at over 90 years old has never eaten anything man made! Still it is vitally important that all of us learn to eat as healthy as possible for the health of our hearts and to have a chance at a longer life.

One thing we know for certain is that if you eat a diet that is high in saturated fats like those found in fatty red meats and cooking oils you are going to see an increase in cholesterol which is proven to be a major factor in heart disease. A recent study that was just released states that just being overweight a few pounds can contribute to heart disease, so you might want to start on that diet and exercise program now! One simple thing that you can do to prevent heart disease is to eat more fish. Salmon, herring and sardines are all excellent sources of Omega 3 essential fatty acids. Many other fish are good for heart health as well, although Omega 3 may help to get your cholesterol down to a healthier level easier. Even red meat lovers can learn to enjoy seafood and nuts for their main sources of protein.

Use monounsaturated fats such as olive oil to protect your heart, olive oil is an ideal choice for cooking, dressing, or even as a dipping sauce. It is also well documented that eating a diet high in fiber will help to control cholesterol. Whole grain products are very high in fiber and also help to control sugar absorption which will go a long way to keeping your digestive system healthy.

Choosing the right carbohydrates is also important for heart health. You need to avoid high sugar food like candy, pastries, cakes and cookies and eat healthy carbohydrates like whole grain bread and pasta, brown rice, and plenty of vegetables. As a matter of fact fruits and vegetables should be the core of a healthy diet. A simple rule of thumb to avoid processed foods is to do your shopping on the outside aisles of the grocery store.

As far as cooking methods go, frying is a total no-no. Stir frying in olive oil or canola oil is okay but you should never deep fry foods and that goes for eating out as well. Chicken is healthy and good for you if you remove the skin and bake the chicken instead of frying.

Making these changes will take time before they become habits but just remember that eating healthy is essential for a healthy heart and a long life.

How To Lower High Cholesterol Levels Naturally

High cholesterol levels can occur as a result of eating too many saturated fats and not enough fibrous foods such as fruits and vegetables and nuts and seeds. It can also result of being overweight or obese and living a sedentary lifestyle, as well as from diseases such as diabetes, high blood pressure, high triglycerides, kidney and liver diseases or an under-active thyroid. Cholesterol is required in the body to help metabolize fat soluble vitamins, as well as to help with the production of certain hormones and bile. However, when the levels become too high, it puts one at risk for certain types of cancers as well as atherosclerosis, stroke, heart attacks and many other cardiovascular diseases. Therefore it is essential to lower high cholesterol levels when they get too high.

Lots of Fruits and Vegetables. Consuming lots of fruits and vegetables will help to lower high cholesterol levels naturally. They are high in fiber, which helps to prevent the absorption of cholesterol in the digestive tract. The soluble fiber binds itself to the cholesterol and other toxins and removes it from the body.

Many fruits and vegetables also contain plant sterols and plant stanols, which work together in a similar manner as prescription drugs to help lower high cholesterol levels. The only difference is that the plant sterols and stanols are natural, and thus they do not cause any harmful side effects that a lot of prescription drugs do.

Foods High in Niacin. High Cholesterol is often treated with higher dosages of a B vitamin, also known as niacin. When given as a drug, it can cause side effects, but niacin can also be obtained from certain plant-based foods in lower dosages and without any side-effects. These foods include almonds and almond butter, peanuts and peanut butter, pecans, pumpkin seeds, sunflower seeds, leafy greens such as kale and spinach, carrots, celery, broccoli, peppers, asparagus and mushrooms.

Foods High in Omega 3 and 6 Fatty Acids. Omega 3 and omega 6 fatty acids have also been shown to lower cholesterol levels naturally. These are fats that can be found in avocados, walnuts, flax seeds and flax seed oil, hemp seeds and pumpkin seeds.

Regular Exercise. Getting the heart rate up at least 3 to 4 times per week can also help to lower high cholesterol levels dramatically. Studies show that those who do not engage in regular exercise are more likely to have high cholesterol levels than those who exercise regularly.

Maintain a Healthy Weight. Excess body weight has also been shown to increase the LDL (bad) cholesterol levels. Regular exercise and a healthy diet will help to maintain a healthy weight, so that the risks can be reduced.

3 Effective Ways To Lower Cholesterol And Prevent Heart Disease

High cholesterol and heart disease have been shown to go hand in hand. It is so important if you have high cholesterol that you lower it as soon as possible. There are many simple things that you can start doing everyday to lower your cholesterol level. This article will show you 3 smart and simple things that you can do:

#1. Eat Whole Grains

How many times have you seen the cheerios commercials that tell you by eating cheerios you can lower your cholesterol? Well they are right! Eating whole grain cereals really can help in lowering cholesterol quite a bit!

#2. Diet and Exercise

I know you probably don't want to hear this but it's true... diet and exercise are a definite way to lower cholesterol. Eating less processed foods and more whole foods is good for you, processed foods are known to raise cholesterol and can cause obesity and heart disease. Whole foods have been known to lower both of these. Getting your 30 to 60 minutes a day of exercise is a fool proof way to get that cholesterol level down and prevent heart disease. Getting exercise will keep your blood sugar level in control and will help you to lose weight. Take a walk or ride a bike. Anything that will get you up and moving can help.

#3. Just say no to saturated fats!

Cutting down on saturated fat will help to lower that high cholesterol. Cutting down on saturated fat means not eating as much butter, oil, etc. None of those foods are good for you.

There are so many other things that you can do to lower cholesterol levels. Consuming more nuts and drinking certain kinds of teas has also been proven to lower cholesterol along with managing your stress levels too. If you doing just a few of these things on a regular basis you will be on your way to a lower cholesterol level.

CHAPTER FOUR
THE RIGHT FOODS FOR ANXIETY AND OTHER MENTAL DISORDERS

Successful people don't always have time to eat well. Busy schedules, new diets, and fast food can keep you from getting proper nutrition. What you might not realize is that not getting proper nutrition could be whats getting you down. There is a known correlation between mental illnesses like anxiety and depression and lack of serotonin in the brain. Another "feel good" chemical that your body can release due to certain foods is endorphins. Even missing melatonin can keep you from getting to sleep at night. Try some of these foods for anxiety and depression and see if they're "just what the doctor ordered."

Serotonin is an important part of signaling in nerve cells in the brain. Lack of serotonin has shown to be a leading cause of depression and anxiety. While there are many drugs out there that can artificially enhance serotonin levels, just eating the right foods can do this as well. The two main building blocks of serotonin are tryptophan and omega 3 fatty acids.

Have you ever felt like going to sleep after a large portion of Thanksgiving turkey? That's the tryptophan at work. Turkey and other meats like lean beef are great sources of tryptophan. Omega 3 fatty acids are the other key ingredient, and as you may well know, fish oil is the most talked about source.

Other foods that you'll find your omega 3's in are eggs, avocados, and flax seeds.

Endorphins are a slightly different character. While not necessary for every day functioning, they're a chemical that your body produces as a painkiller and sedative. You may have heard of a "runner's high." This is the body's response to the stresses of strenuous exercise by producing endorphins. Fortunately, you can generate endorphins from the food you eat as well. Dark Chocolate is a great food for both endorphins and serotonin. But, this does tend to be a temporary high. Another way to stimulate endorphin production is to eat hot and spicy foods. Your brain can be tricked into thinking your mouth is on fire and needs the endorphins to kill the pain.

Does your anxiety keep you up at night? Try some sunflower seeds before you go to bed. Sunflower seeds are a great source of melatonin, believed to be an important factor in deep sleep. Other good sources of melatonin are sour cherries, fennel seeds, alfalfa sprouts, and coriander seeds.

Changing your diet can have a very deep impact in reducing your anxiety attacks. Combining the food for anxiety relief with daily exercise will not only help reduce anxiety, it also puts you on track for a healthier life. That is because eating the right food for anxiety will help maintain the proper function of the brain, giving you better control over stress. It will also give you more energy, taking away the ill effects of depression and excess nervous energy.

So how does a proper diet come into play when dealing with anxiety?

It is important to note that all living cells are continuously subject to imperfect nutrition. The brain cells likewise, gets its nutrition from blood, which in turn gets its nutrients from the food you eat each day. Malnutrition therefore weakens the brain to handle any excess mental stress that goes along with the proper function of your overall body performance.

Note that an improper diet can cause the body to produce excess adrenaline that normally results in an anxiety attack when it does not get switch off.

Some of the food for anxiety that contains minerals that the body needs to function properly are:

1. Magnesium: Plays an important role in relation to blood pressure by ensuring proper blood vessel relaxation and contraction, thus maintaining a proper heart. Magnesium contributes to the electrical activity of the brain thereby affecting the proper running of nerve conduction as well as muscle contraction.

Try eating leafy vegetables, barley and whole grains which contains a healthy dosage of magnesium.

2. Vitamin B: The B vitamins are responsible for proper function of the nervous system. They have been found to stabilize the lactate levels of the body, which are responsible for the anxiety attacks.

Turkey, chicken, sunflower seeds, spinach, broccoli, avocados and yogurts are contains are good sources of the B vitamins.

3. Calcium: They are needed for normal communication among nerve cells as well as muscle contraction which supports the body during anxiety. Dietary calcium may also help in lowering blood pressure, which may raise during anxiety.

Some good source of calcium includes tofu, soybeans and broccoli.

4. Vitamin C: The C Vitamin is responsible for the creation and maintenance of the hormone Cortisol which has an important role in stress levels. As Vitamin C contains anti-oxidants, it also provides a more effective stress coping mechanisms.

Some sources of the C Vitamin includes Oranges, grapefruit, tomatoes and berries.

Some of the food that you should avoid:

1. Alcohol: These not only robs the body of magnesium, but also dehydrates and cause nervousness and irritability.

2. Coffee: Caffeine can deplete the body of magnesium, making you feel nervous and jittery. Yes, that includes fizzy drinks.

3. Processed food: These may be heavy in pesticides, harmful unsaturated fats and additives, which kills the beneficial bacteria needed to absorb the nutrients from the food you take.

4. Sugars: Sugar gives you the swings from high to low blood sugar and can result in corresponding mood swings. Therefore, if possible, try avoiding it.

Taking the right food for anxiety will improve your overall function of the brain and body, giving them a stronger counter in reacting against response malfunction thereby reducing the anxiety attacks frequency.

Eating For Anxiety

Anxiety is an issue for so many people and learning ways to reduce the symptoms naturally is always helpful. People with who deal with it know how frustrating it can be to feel high stress levels as well as dealing with panic attacks. Diet may help in reducing the symptoms by eating the right foods and avoiding ones that may increase symptoms.

Three things to avoid most include caffeine, refined sugar, and alcohol. While you may not want to give these up completely, cutting back on them may help with mood. Caffeine for example can cause that jittery feeling as well as interrupting sleep.

Alcohol may feel good in the beginning but the after effects can cause anxiety-like symptoms.

The food that helps include plenty of water, foods rich in antioxidants, vegetables, fruit, nuts, and seeds. Avoid processed food as much as possible as these can be high in refined sugar and sodium. It can be difficult to eat enough of the right foods on a regular basis so considering a nutritional supplement may help. A good multivitamin may be enough to supplement nutritional needs. Besides eating for anxiety, other natural options include breathing properly. Deep belly breathing is a great way to calm yourself. Whenever I feel high levels of anxiety, I do deep belly breathing and it helps to keep my symptoms under control. This helps a lot, especially when you are worried about panic attacks.

10 Foods For Treating Anxiety

Anxiety disorder can cause big disturbance in your everyday living. It badly influences your disposition in life. The nervous tension that anxiety brings can drag you down, and even push you into drug and alcohol addiction. It is normal to feel anxious every now and then, but if the reason behind your anxious feeling is not very sensible, then there might be something wrong with you. The good news is that anxiety disorders can be treated and avoided. Nevertheless, it must be treated right away in order for you to steer clear of breakdowns and other serious personality abnormalities.

There are many things that can help you cope up with anxiety. One thing that can help you get rid of anxiety is to have a balanced, healthy diet. Fortunately, there are many foods that can aid you with your anxiety disorder. If you want to get back that hale and hearty living, you should consider adding these 10 foods for treating anxiety to your diet.

Honey is considered as a miracle food. It has natural contents that are good for health. Aside from its delicious taste, honey has been widely used in medicine. If you have anxiety, consuming about two tablespoons of honey a day can help regulate your body and make your thinking clearer.

Fish is rich in Vitamin B3 or niacin, which is the vitamin that promotes the creation of serotonin. Serotonin is a neurotransmitter that is responsible for giving a person a well-balanced mind. Aside from niacin, fish is also rich with oils and fats that are good for the heart.

Mushroom has excellent Vitamin B5 or pantothenic acid contents. This nutrient supports the adrenal glands in the body. Foods rich in pantothenic acid like mushrooms will also improve the body's response to stress.

Oranges are rich in Vitamin C. Vitamin C or ascorbic acid produces corsitol hormone which is responsible for maintaining stress levels. Another good thing about oranges, and other similar foods, is that it is rich in anti-oxidants.

Liver and other organ meats are rich in Vitamin A. Eating this kind of foods will make you have a better stress coping mechanism.

Berries, particularly blueberries and acacia berries are super foods for anxiety. They regulate blood sugar levels and improve brain function. Berries are also said to help illnesses such as cancer and Alzheimer's disease.

Almonds have the ability to enhance mood because they are rich in Vitamin B12 and zinc. It also improves immune system and helps the body fight heart disease.

Sunflower seeds are rich in Vitamin E. Aside from the many skin benefits that you can get from this nutrient; you can also have more protection from free radicals. It can also regulate your mood because this kind of food improves cell communication.

Peaches have phytonutrients and natural sedative contents. Eating peaches can alleviate stress and even help fight cancer.

Green leafy vegetables have high amount of magnesium. When you are anxious, your magnesium level is low. Eating green leafy vegetables can bring back magnesium and other essential nutrients to your body.

When you eat these foods and consume the right amount of vitamins and minerals, you will have more defenses against anxiety and other disorders. Keep in mind that the first step to a better living is strengthening your mind and body.

Avoiding Mental Disorders Through The Aid Of Vitamins And Minerals

When we think about the benefits of being ensuring a good bill of health by keeping track of our daily intake of prescribed vitamins, minerals and as well as the other nutrients that are needed by your body in order to stay healthy.

It is important to be conscious of the fact that deficiencies in the daily intake of vitamins and minerals can negatively affect not only your physical capabilities but your how your mind functions as well. Recent research has indicated that such deficiencies can even contribute to one of the most common mental illnesses of all, depression.

The Vitamin B complex is incredibly important to our mental well-being and functioning. Even relatively small deficiencies can have an adverse effect on a person's mental health over time. While serious nutrient deficiencies can actually contribute to serious mental illnesses. As for the case of trying your best to avoid mental illnesses, it is highly important to make sure that your daily diet meets the recommended amount of the Vitamin B complex.

It is also interesting to note that those with alcohol problems - often used as a way to cope up with depression can actually worsen one's situation, are often suffering from Vitamin B complex deficiencies. This is because alcohol actually destroys the Vitamin B in a person's body.

A lack of thiamine can also lead to a lack of energy as well as to being sluggish all the time. When ignored and not taken care of immediately, it can actually lead to deep fatigue, anxiety, depression and even to having suicidal tendencies. It can also bring on insomnia, which can contribute to the worsening of each and every one of these symptoms. Serious deficiency in niacin has been clinically associated with various mental symptoms like cognitive slowness which concerns the processing of information, dementia, anxiety and psychosis. Vitamin B5 has been found to play a big role in the formation of hormones as well as other brain chemical processes that are related to a person's mood. Nutritional deficiencies can lead to stress and certain types of depression. Vitamin B6 is essential to the production of serotonin and dopamine. If continuously ignored, the lack of Vitamin B12 can eventually lead to various mental disorders such as serious mood swings, mania, paranoia, dementia and even hallucinations.

Vitamin C is also important in the prevention or easing the state of depression that a person is in. It is important to note that many common medications, both over the counter and prescription drugs, can actually rob the body of Vitamin C, which is why a lot of doctors tend to add vitamin C supplements alongside their anti-depressant prescriptions.

Deficiencies in a number of minerals have been highly associated with depression and other mental disorders. Among these are magnesium, calcium, iron, zinc, potassium and manganese. They actually all combine in order to produce and release serotonin and other compounds that can have positive effects on a person's mood and mental health.

Other symptoms of a poor mental health which are greatly associated with deficiencies in the essential minerals that a person needs, include paranoia, confusion, anxiety, depression, fatigue and tearfulness.

The brain is ruled by the chemical interactions that obviously take place within it. These chemicals have a delicate balance to maintain and nutrition definitely plays an integral role both in the formation of these essential chemicals and their proper maintenance. On every level of mental mood and functioning, it is absolutely necessary that we make sure to meet the recommended daily intake levels of vitamins, minerals as well as the other nutrients. Dietary supplements, when used according to recommended dosages, are a safe means of seeing to it that our minds are functioning properly and effectively.

Top 10 Greatest Anti Anxiety Foods For Anxiety Sufferers

Isn't diet a confusing thing? Add the fact that people who suffer from chronic anxiety and panic disorder have difficulty getting through a day filled with over worry and panic, and you've got a person stuck in constant confusion and frustration on how to deal with their anxiety. Many researchers have proven the positive connections between consuming the proper foods, and combating anxiety naturally.

So let's get to the top 10 anti anxiety foods on the planet you must add to your diet consistently to combat chronic anxiety:

1) Sushi - Don't like fish? Well it's time to turn that ship around starting today! Sushi is loaded with stress relieving properties such as magnesium and vitamin B2 just to name a few. Time to take your loved one out for a night of sushi!

2) Blueberries - These little blue guys are loaded with antioxidants and vitamin C, which are both incredible stress busters and will help with dealing with anxiety. Best advice I can give you is to throw some blueberries into your morning shake, sit back, and reap the benefits.

3) Greek Yogurt - Get some plain, unsweetened Greek yogurt if you want to lower your blood pressure and get a great big dose of vitamins B6 and B12. Greek yogurt also contains magnesium and calcium all great anxiety fighters. Opa!

4) Almonds - OK, you have no excuses when it comes to eating almonds. The best thing I did as I worked on ending my own 6-year struggle with panic and anxiety was to replace my bag a day potato chip eating habit, with a handful of almonds in my pocket everyday. Go raw over roasted almonds and avoid the salted versions as sodium contributes to high blood pressure, which escalates feelings of panic and anxiety quickly.

5) Peppermint Tea - I can add teas to the list of anxiety fighter's right? Talking purely from experience here, I found peppermint tea to be better for anxiety then chamomile tea and helped me keep my focus for longer periods, as well as kept my performance up (in every way possible). The scent of it, the taste of it, everything that comes with peppermint tea is awesome. If you feel that caffeine in tea doesn't work well for dealing with your anxiety, you can always get the caffeine-free version. Time for a cup-o-tea!

6) Oatmeal - Depleted Serotonin levels can increase anxiety levels and keep you agitated for long periods of time, that's where oatmeal comes in. Eating foods rich in fiber (whole grain carbohydrates) will get a steady flow of serotonin working for you. Other rich in fiber carbs to keep in mind are quinoa, and whole wheat bread.

7) Turkey - Thanksgiving Day should be the best day for anyone suffering from panic and constant anxiety. Why you may ask? Turkey contains an essential amino acid known as tryptophan, which eases anxiety and calms the mind. Think back to those days when you felt 'nappy' after a big turkey dinner, that's the tryptophan talking.

8) Beets - Time to get that old juicer out and start making some fresh beet juice! With the amazing anti-inflammatory properties that come with fresh beet juice, you can't afford not to make this the #1 juicing vegetable for your mind and body, as you work towards stopping your anxiety naturally.

9) Ginger - Hate eating ginger by itself? Throw it in your blender with blueberries and some leafy greens! Ginger contains an antioxidant called Gingerol, which gets rid of those bad chemicals roaming around your body that usually leads to mental and physical stress and anxiety. Still don't want to throw it in your blender to make juice out of it? Fine, there are many herbal teas that ginger is diffused in. Gingerize yourself to help stop anxiety naturally.

10) Broccoli - Time to re train those yucky memories of broccoli from when you were a kid. Broccoli is absolutely packed with vitamins that include stress and anxiety fighting essential B vitamins, and folic acid (a family member for B vitamins). If you're looking to relieve anxiety and stress and even send away any of those depressive symptoms you may be having, it's time to regularly add broccoli to your diet.

You may be thinking, how can I possibly add all these foods to my anti anxiety diet all of a sudden. That's where planning and patience comes in. The great thing is you don't need loads of each and every anti anxiety food to feel the benefits, small amounts of daily intake will make a huge difference in the short tern, and your mind and body will thank you for it.

Living With Anxiety: Food and Anxiety, A Love/Hate Relationship

Living with Anxiety has allowed me to rediscover food and get back in the direction of healthy eating. By "healthy eating", I do not imply good for my figure or for my body, no, I mean good for a "healthy" mental. That latter statement was made true by my very own recovery from anxiety.

When Food Was My Enemy

My excessive caffeine intake was not haphazard, it was planned and systematic. I wanted to fill my stomach with something other than food, because I did not want to put on weight. Yes, vanity almost cost me my mental health! When I changed my job, I went from a highly active position to a more sedentary one, which as you may guess took a toll on my figure. I felt like I was putting on the pounds and I even could feel my derriere expanding. Needless to say that my reaction was completely irrational and unrealistic, but it became an obsession. I became self conscious of my weight and decided to take action. I am not one to take pills, so diet pills was never an option, but I wanted something that would show fast results in combination with a workout regimen. So it was that I turned to caffeine.

The plan was simple; substituting food with a caffeinated beverage would work perfectly well because caffeine can curb my appetite and keep me alert and energized at the same time.

The perfect diet plan!! I designed that plan based on what I saw on magazines and on TV. For example, have you ever noticed that movie stars are always seen holding a cup of Joe (black and no sugar, I am sure), even coming out of their workout session? How unhealthy!! I did not care about "unhealthy", I cared about keeping my silhouette. I was hooked and blindly (or stupidly) took the path that led to my demise.

And The Dice Was Cast

So a typical day with that diet went as follows. I would have a zillion cups of caffeinated beverages (a Vivanno strengthened with a shot of espresso from Starbucks and black tea in a tea bag) for breakfast and no food. Then at lunch, I would alternate between eating a sandwich or a can of diet coke with some cookies (yes, I was definitely delusional!!). Finally, dinner would comprise a regular meal or, on occasion, a cup of black tea and a chocolate bar.

That diet worked well for me since I did not put on weight. Indeed, regardless of the kind of food that I was eating, I was eating less overall and it was the reduced quantity that made the difference.

I was so absorbed with my looks that I did not worry when other changes began to show. For example, I was becoming very impatient with everything and anything. It was so severe that even watching a movie was difficult because I just wanted to skip some parts. My concentration was very poor, as I found myself distracted quite often. Last but not least, I began to feel overwhelmed by things. That was a phenomenon that should have set off the alarm, but I did nothing about it because it was only transient. I recall one night feeling extremely overwhelmed by some work that I had to do; I felt dizzy and hot and was slightly hyperventilating. I remember that at that point I had to reassure myself and rationalize the situation before the feeling dissipated. Ironically, I had my first panic attack two days later. In the psychological jargon, those symptoms would be called prodromes, because they were early symptoms indicating the onset of an anxiety attack.

It did not become clear to me right away that eating healthy was going to help me recover from my anxiety, but as I researched online easy ways of controlling anxiety it became evident that it was paramount to a long-term recovery.

Food for Thoughts

The brain is a glutton. It hoards 15% to 20% of the total glucose (fuel for cells) produced in the body, which means that a large part of what you eat fuels your brain. It is well-known that malnutrition leads to a slew of physical problems, but the psychological consequences are somehow less emphasized. One such consequence is the impact of undernourishment on moods. For example, anorexic individuals almost always display labile moods marked by negative and depressive thoughts. That is not just hunger causing those mood problems but also the fact that the brain does not receive sufficient nutrients to function well. Other times a sick brain requires a specific diet to work properly as is the case with anxiety. That is the reason that mental health professionals recommend a diet rich in protein and low in carbohydrates in combination with therapy to help relieve anxiety symptoms.

In my case, it was clear that caffeine triggered my anxiety attack but a fact that was less obvious to me was that poor nutrition undoubtedly exacerbated the problem. Interestingly, I was quite moody during that time period, and I was often afflicted with negative moods. In turn the negative moods increased my anxiety, so once again I was caught up in a vicious cycle.

Once it was clear to me that I had to change my diet, I established a specific eating pattern that was going to be my most efficient weapon against anxiety.

Eating Right Became my Biggest Challenge

I felt so good about my plan that I became optimistic about my ability to know what to do about anxiety, but I did not know yet that it was going to be a big hurdle. Indeed as my anxiety reached the full-blown level, I had lost control over my body and, as one of the consequences, I was no longer able to eat. My appetite was very poor (if not non-existent) but I also was not able to swallow food anymore. The following pattern repeated itself during eating.

First, my throat would constrict, making it harder to pass down my esophagus, and finally when food reached my stomach it would trigger a nauseated feeling that simply forced me to stop eating. As a result, I ate considerably less than I should and lost weight. Another irony was that I was losing the weight that was the motivating factor behind my unhealthy eating habit! However, the weight loss was so dramatic and so quick that it made me extremely uncomfortable and worried. In fact when I started to weigh myself on the scale, I realized that I had lost more than 8 pounds in less than two weeks. I could no longer fit in my clothes, but I had no control over it anymore; it was as if I was shedding the pounds by the day. I felt like I was disintegrating.

After a brief moment of depression over my weight loss, I decided to take actions and not let anxiety control my life. The plan of attack required constancy and patience, because it was going to be a slow process. First I had to make sure to have some food for breakfast, regardless of the quantity, because that was to set the tone for the rest of the day. I opted for a PBJ sandwich (peanut butter and jelly sandwich) on a whole grain toast because it was nutritious (protein for strength and natural sugars for alertness) and tasty.

Even though I could not finish the toast, the fact that it tasted good induced me to eat a little bit more every time.

As a matter of fact, taste was going to be my most powerful weapon against the anxiety assault on my body because even tough my physical hunger was somehow stifled, my psychological hunger could only grow. In other words, eating a tasty meal makes you want more of it even if you are already satisfied, because psychologically you are seeking more of that feel-good taste. In eating as in sex, the same pleasure centers are activated in the brain, and as a result eating is physically and psychologically satisfying.

Lunch and dinner were complete meals accompanied with vegetables. I did not eat sandwiches or to go meals, because I wanted to make sure that I ate a balanced diet. Here again taste was important. I selected meals based on my favorite dishes, such as pasta, to ensure that I was going to want to eat despite the nauseating sensations. In addition, I had orange juice all day and I made sure to drink a glass of milk everyday to prevent further weight loss.

I realized later on that liquids were swallowed more easily than food, so there were times when I had the protein shake Ensure and others when I had different kinds of fruit juices.

As time went on this regimen proved successful as I slowly regained a normal appetite. I have to add that meditation is what allowed me to be so mindful of myself and my body, which then helped me resolve the eating issue. Meditation for anxiety was a first-step before my recovery from anxiety.

" Food is for eating, and good food is to be enjoyed "

CHAPTER FIVE
FOODS FOR PREVENT HEART ATTACKS AND STROKES

Heart disease is one of those medical conditions that you need to try and prevent happening rather than try to cure it after it has affected your life. There are several different reasons for heart disease occurring in your body and most of these can be prevented if you lead a healthy lifestyle. Drinking, smoking and a poor diet can all contribute to heart disease and trying to cut these things out of your daily lifestyle is essential.

If you cannot stop them completely then you need to try and cut back and ensure that you exercise daily. High cholesterol is a major factor behind heart disease and you need to maintain a healthy level of this. You should eat a diet which is low in fats and high in fiber. Although you may think this is hard to do, there are many foods which you can eat which are excellent for you. You also need to maintain your weight at a healthy level which will help to keep your heart healthy.

You should try to do at least 30 minutes of exercise per day which can help to reduce the risk of heart disease. Any form of exercise is better than none at all and whether you prefer to take a brisk walk or a run, this will all help you to remain healthy and fit. Exercise doesn't need to be boring and the more fun you can make it, the more likely you are to stick to it. Try to get your family involved in the exercise plan and this will help them to lead a healthy lifestyle as well. If you can make small changes to your lifestyle and encourage your children to lead a healthier life then this will help them in the future.

There are supplements and some foods which you can eat every day which can help your heart to perform better. Vitamin B and C are both excellent for you and can be found in many different foods. Fish oil is also very good for your heart. Including these into your daily diet will help you to ensure that your heart is working well. If you cannot find these vitamins in their natural forms, then taking them as supplements is just as effective. Although you should try to cut out all bad foods including sugar, fats and processed foods, moderation is the key if you are finding this too difficult.

Let's face it, cardiovascular disease, or heart disease, is the number 1 killer in America. Men have a greater tendency to develop heart-related diseases, but each year, more and more women are experiencing this condition.

For the prevention and treatment of cardiovascular diseases, several natural substances have been studied and found to be effective. Before you start on any natural form of treatment, though, make sure you first consult with your physician and obtain approval and constant supervision.

Natural Ways to prevent heart disease

Vitamin C improves the dilation of blood vessels in atherosclerotic patients and those affected by congestive heart failure and high blood pressure.

Vitamin B Complex breaks down homocysteine for improved heart performance.

CoQ10, when taken in combination with Vitamin E, has been found to help treat heart disease.

Fish oils have been found to reduce the risk of arrhythmia, atrial fibrillation, and heart palpitations.

Why Omega-3 fatty acids are so popular? Omega-3 fatty acids from fish oils and mussels have earned the nod of hundreds of health professionals in recent years because of their role in the management and prevention of heart diseases. Since the 1970s, there has been significant interest in the role of Omega-3 polyunsaturated fatty acids (PUFAs) due to the convincing results of several lab studies. One such study was made by Dyerberg and Bang on Greenland Eskimos. They found that these people had a lower incidence of death resulting from coronary heart disease, as compared to the Danes who lived on a "western" diet.

This, despite the fact that their diet was rich in fat (seal fat, mainly). After studying the results, they concluded that it was mainly the Eskimos' diet, which was rich in Omega-3 PUFAs, that caused reduced thrombosis tendencies and increased vessel dilation.

Good Eating Habits Can Prevent Heart Disease - Know What To Eat, What To Avoid, And How To Cook

You can prevent heart disease to a great extent just by improving your eating habits. So, educate yourself about the food items that you should eat and the ones that you have to avoid. Besides that, it will also be great if you learn how to cook a heart healthy diet. You will find the following information very helpful in this regard.

Eat Right Foods

Following is a list of food items that you should include in your diet to prevent heart disease.

- Use unsaturated vegetable oils, such as sunflower, safflower, olive, and canola.

- You need 6 cooked ounces of protein food group on a daily basis. Peas and beans can be good source of protein.

- Your daily food intake must also include 2-4 servings of dairy products. However, you are recommended to eat low-fat or nonfat milk. You can also try yogurt.

- Include plenty of whole grains in your diet, such as pasta, rice, and cereal. Eat at least 6 servings of these food items on a daily basis.

- Most importantly, you must eat at least 5-6 servings of fresh vegetables and fruits.

Food Items That You Have To Avoid

Following is a brief rundown about the food items that you have to avoid in order to prevent heart disease.

- Goose and duck meat should be avoided at all costs.

- Cut down the intakes of high-fat processed meats, such as sausage, bologna, and hot dogs.

- The use of organ meats should also be taken in a very limited quantity. Organ meats may include brain, kidney, sweetbreads, and liver of chicken or other birds or animals.

- High-fat dairy products should top your avoid list. Such products include cheese, butter, ice cream, cream, and whole milk.

Some Heart Healthy Cooking Tips

In order to keep your heart healthy and to prevent heart disease, you should also be very careful while cooking the different food items. Following are some quick tips.

- If you must eat meat, make sure that you have trimmed fat thoroughly. If you are cooking poultry, don't forget to remove its skin before cooking.

- For basting, you can use marinade, fruit juice, and wine.

- Use very low amount of solid fats (if at all you have to use it) while cooking. Solid fats include soft margarine, lard, and shortening (fat that is used to make pastries).

- You should try cooking methods that require no or very little fat. Such cooking methods may include broiling, baking, and boiling.

- When browning, you are recommended to use a cooking rack to drain off fat.

- Don't use the yolk of the eggs in your recipes. But, you can use egg whites.

Overall, the basic idea is to eat from every food group - you just have to focus on the quantity, quality, and the amount of fat and salt in it. In order to prevent heart disease, you should eat foods that are low in salt and fat.

How To Prevent Heart Disease with Diet

Anything that serves to damage the inner lining of blood vessels and impedes the transportation of oxygen and nutrition to the heart can be defined as a risk of heart disease. Most heart diseases are preventable with a change of life style and healthy diet. Unhealthy diet is a major cause of heart diseases resulting in the buildup of cholesterol and fat in the inner wall of arteries that narrows the arteries, impedes the circulation and eventually causes heart attacks.

To prevent heart diseases, your daily diet should contain:

1. Fiber - Fiber can be soluble or insoluble. Soluble fiber can lower your LDL and raise your HDL cholesterol while insoluble fiber has no effect on cholesterol but promotes regular bowel movements. The intake of fatty foods causes the liver to release bile into the intestines to break down the fat. The soluble fiber will help eliminate the bile instead of returning it to the blood resulting in reduced amounts of cholesterol in the blood.

2. Reduce intake of saturated fat and trans fat - We know that saturated and trans fat are toxins causing cholesterol to build up in the arteries damaging the arterial wall and narrows the arterial passage in result of poor circulation and oxygen transportation to our body in result of high blood pressure as the heart has to work harder than normal in order to provide enough nutrition to the body's cells. Eventually, the heart will fail and result in heart diseases. It is recommended that you reduce the intake of animal fat and increase the intake of cold water fish which is the best sources of omega 3 and 6 fatty acids that can help your cholesterol levels as well as lowering your blood pressure.

3. Diet high in complex carbohydrates - Vegetables, fruits, some beans and grains contain high amounts of plant pigments known as flavonoids that provide healthy protection against heart diseases. Unfortunately study shows that diets high in complex carbohydrate may increase the release of too much insulin to respond to carbohydrates in the diet. The type and amount of carbohydrate foods may need individual monitoring. Please consult with your doctor if you wish to include high amounts of complex carbohydrates in your diet.

4. Drink half of your body weight of water or juices in ounces - If you weigh 160 pounds then you are require to drink 80 ounces of water or juices to prevent the cells in our body to become dehydrated. Maintaining normal function of our body's cells is a healthy way to normalize high blood pressure.

Preventing heart disease isn't as hard as you think it is. There are 3 simple things that you can do everyday to lower your risk.

#1. Eat Right

Diet is so important when it comes to preventing heart disease. What you eat has a very big effect on you and if you are eating the wrong kinds of food your risk for heart disease go up.

Avoiding processed and greasy, fatty foods can do your heart so much good. Instead of eating the unhealthy foods, try eating more whole foods.

Whole foods are foods that are close to their natural form, they have not been processed and stripped of the nutrients. This includes fruits, vegetables, whole grains, and some forms of dairy. By eating these healthier foods you will lower cholesterol which lowers your risk for heart disease. Next time you go to the store avoid all the aisles with processed and fatty foods. Doing this will help you to resist the temptation of buying unhealthy food.

#2. Exercise Regularly

Most people cringe when the hear that they need to start exercising regularly, but you don't have to be scared of it! This doesn't mean that you need to go run 10 miles everyday or climb to the top of a mountain. Simply taking your dog on a walk or riding your bike on a nice bike trail is good enough. Playing a small game of soccer with your kids in the backyard is a great way to keep them entertained and get the exercise you need. Anything that gets you up and moving is a great start to regular exercise.

#3. Set Goals

Go see your doctor and find out where you need to be as far as your heart health goes. Once you know, set up a plan to get there. Set up a certain amount of time that you have to reach your goal and then plan out how you will do it. Start out with simple things that can easily be done on a regular basis then work your way up from there. Setting goals for yourself is such a great way to get yourself motivated.

Therefore, in order to lower the risk of heart diseases foods consumed in everyday diet become one of many important factors. Here are some foods that I have found can actually lower high blood pressure and levels of cholesterol resulting in lowering the risk of heart diseases.

1. **Fresh water algae.** Fresh water algae contains chlorophyIl-rich foods that is a powerful antioxidant for protection of build up of free radicals and restoring DNA of damaged cells. It also contains high amounts of Omega 3 and 6 fatty acids that can help to maintain normal blood pressure as well as cholesterol levels. Omega 3 and 6 fatty acids also inhibit blood clotting that causes the blockage of arteries and heart diseases.

2. **Onions and garlic.** Garlic and onions contain high amounts of sulfur compounds that not only help to improve circulation of blood but also help to keep your platelets from clumping together. Daily consumption of both garlic and onions help to keep blood pressure and cholesterol levels in healthy range. Be sure to talk to your doctor if you are taking any blood thinner medicines.

3. **Nuts and seeds.** Nuts and seeds contain high amounts of unsaturated fat and vitamin E. Unsaturated fat helps to prevent clots of arteries and lower cholesterol levels. Vitamin E, and the antioxidants beta varotene on the other hand stops bad cholesterol LDL from building up in the arteries, decreasing the risk of heart attacks.

4. **Vegetables and fruits.** Vegetable and fruits contain high amounts vitamins A, E, C and B. Vitamin E, the antioxidants beta carotene and vitamin C help to strengthen your small blood vessels and thins your blood so it can flow smoothly in result of lowering the risk of heart disease and strokes. Plums, tomatoes, and watercress are the best choices.

There are many more foods that can help to lower high blood pressure and cholesterol levels such as horsenut, grape juices, and apples.

Take care of your body it's the only place you have to live

Jim Rohn

CHAPTER SIX
OTHER REMEDIES TO LIVE A
HEALTHIER LIFESTYLE

It is a proven fact that people who engage in regular physical activity lead healthier lives than those who do not. Adding even a moderate amount of physical activity to your routine can make drastic difference in your lifestyle. You might start with something very simple, such as taking the stairs instead of the elevator or going for a short walk on your lunch break. Eventually, it is good to work up to the point where you are getting 30 minutes or more of cardiovascular exercise at least three times a week. Here are some of the benefits of physical activities.

1. Mental and Emotional Benefits: Getting regular exercise can improve your thinking and your moods. It will help you be more alert, be happier, and have more energy. You will experience a high right after your workout, and the good feelings will sustain themselves in between workouts.

2. Physical Benefits: There are many physical benefits to exercise. It is good for your heart, and helps to prevent heart disease. It helps you maintain a healthy weight, and therefore helps to fight diseases that are common with obesity, such as diabetes. It makes your muscles stronger, and helps your lungs to function better.

3. Appearance: Getting regular exercise helps your appearance in all kinds of ways. It helps to tone your muscles, so you appear healthier and fitter. It makes your skin softer and firmer, and helps to fight skin problems such as acne. It makes your eyes brighter, and the mental and emotional benefits often manifest themselves in your appearance.

These are just some of the benefits of physical activities. If you begin to incorporate exercise into your daily life, you will notice all kinds of other benefits for yourself. The heightened energy level itself can lead to all sorts of positive changes.

How To Benefit From Regular Exercise At Any Age

Benefits of exercise can be reaped at any age provided you are regular with your routine. Regular exercise no matter what it is can be and has proved to be beneficial in various ways. If you are not a gym person or you hate doing aerobics you can choose what gives you pleasure. Remember the idea is to lead an active life and not a sedentary one.

Here are the ten benefits of regular exercise which can be anything that suits you or the one that you enjoy the most and thus leading an active life.

1. **Reduced bone loss.** As you age your bones starts losing its tissues, this process is known as osteoporosis. Osteoporosis can increase the risk of fracture, as your bones become brittle and can easily break. Regular exercise helps you build the bone tissues, thus reducing the risk of osteoporosis. Diabetic and women are at more risk of osteoporosis.

2. **Decreased risk of cardiovascular diseases.** Regular exercise can also reduce the risk of heart attack and other cardiovascular disease. It also helps in fighting cholesterol. Regular exercise can also help you fight your blood pressure problems.

3. **Weight loss and maintenance.** Proper diet and exercise can help you shed those extra kilos from your body, better still it will help you maintain that new slim and svelte look.

4. **Increased mental focus.** With regular exercise children can increase their concentration power and elderly people can stall the memory loss problems common to their age. Increased mental focus keeps you agile and healthy for a long time.

5. **Increased energy.** Do you feel tired all the time? Do you feel that you have no energy left in your body? Well with regular exercise you will feel rejuvenated and filled with new energy.

Exercise boost the blood circulation thus making you feel energised and fresh.

6. **Increased stamina.** If you dread going to shopping because the bags are too heavy for you, then exercising is your answer. Exercising regularly not only keeps you fit but also helps to boost your stamina, thus making most of the day to day jobs easier for you.

7. **Promotes better sleep.** Having troubled in sleeping? Or are you not able to sleep deeply? Fret not. Start exercising and you will feel that you are not only sleeping better but also feeling fresh in the morning. Ready to face any challenge that life throws at you with a smile.

8. **Increased intimacy.** Add a sparkle to your sex life with regular exercise. As you age you either tend to lose interest in sex or you start becoming conscious of your looks. With the regular physical activity you will be able to add a sparkle to your forgotten sex life.

9. **Beats stress.** Beat the stress with regular physical activity. Office tensions, family obligations put a stress on you which can only be overcome by regular physical activity. Exercising releases a brain chemical that uplifts your mood and helps you calm down.

10. **Suppresses depression.** Are you depressed? Hit to the gym, or do some gardening or go for a long walk. Chances are that when you are done with you will feel relaxed, happy, and no more depressed.

These are just few of the benefits of regular exercise but there are many more such benefits. So start exercising and stop being lazy.

Benefit Of Eating Less

Nowadays, more and more people are trying to reduce their calories intake. How much we eat does not affect only our looks, but our health as well. It seems that people who eat less have a lower risk of heart disease, less chances of having a stroke or getting diabetes.

Moreover, some even believe that eating less will extend their life span and will help them avoid health problems associated with aging. Some researchers calculated that (based on tests conducted on animals) every calorie we avoid means about 30 seconds extra life.

The "French paradox" is a very good example for this matter. Only 7% of French people are obese (as compared to more than 22% of all Americans) although they do not eat only salads all day. French people, like every one else, like to smoke, drink wine, eat food products high in calories (buttered croissants, goose livers, pastries, etc.). The only difference is that they eat less of everything as they are used to serving smaller portions.

Researchers found that an average food portion in Paris has about 270 g, while in Philadelphia an average food portion has about 350g, an American hot dog is about 60% larger that a French one, a soft drink is 52% larger in US as compared to France, etc.

As sometimes we may find it difficult to reduce and sustain the intake of calories, I thought that presenting some tricks might help us reduce the quantity of food we eat and prevail in the battle with calories would be helpful.

1. Eat less, but more often. Is better to eat smaller portions than few large ones because in this way food is properly digested and nutrients are better used. When we eat much, the body cannot effectively "process" all the food.

2. Drink water before you eat. This will make you feel full and will decrease your appetite.

3. Eat in smaller plates. The main advantage of a smaller plate is that it gives the impression of a normal serving although it holds less food. When going to a restaurant switch the dinner plate with a salad one, which is smaller.

4. Brush your teeth. Some people might refuse to have a quick snack or even a meal when their teeth have just been brushed and feel clean.

5. Include more vegetables in your meal. Eating more vegetables can make us fell satiated even if few calories are assimilated. So, look in your meal for ingredients that can be substituted with vegetables.

6. Count calories intake. First of all, it will help you keep track of how many calories have you assimilated during the day and how you can allocate the remaining ones for future meals. Secondly, it might motivate you to reduce the number of calories assimilated daily. You can also practice this when going out for groceries in order to purchase "lighter food products".

7. No more sugar. Sugar is a very important source of calories, causing an increase in appetite. In g of sugar there are approximately 400 calories. Try to replace as much as possible products containing sugar with sugar-free similar products (e.g. replace soft drinks with sugar-free juices, still water, etc.).

8. Eat slower. The body must have time to process and fully estimate the quantity of food that is eaten. When we eat fast, we sometimes might not realize that we are satiated.

9. Say NO to chips, snacks, breads, etc. Besides the fact that such products are well know for their "weight attraction" due to their ingredients, such products can make us want to eat and drinks more (especially salted ones).

10. Chew gum. Chewing sugar-free gum can give us the impression that we are eating. So, when hunger strikes, try first some gum.

11. Avoid foods cooked in oil. Although sometimes fried means tasty, we should bear in mind that oil has a lot of fats and calories (there are more than 100 calories in a spoon of oil). Try to eat as much as possible baked, barbecued foods.

12. Avoid snacks. You will eat less if you have a normal meal as compared to having several snacks before or after meals. So, try to impose a fix schedule in terms of meals.

13. Go for more taste and less quantity. Try to keep as long as you can the taste of something you want to eat in your mouth. For example, if you freeze chocolate, it will melt more slowly in your mouth and you will fell like you have eaten more.

Health Benefits of Drinking Alkaline Water

Water is good for us and as a matter of fact, we are supposed to drink at least 8 glasses of water every day to keep ourselves hydrated and healthy. However not all water is the same and some have more benefits than others, such as drinking alkaline water. First of all drinking alkaline water is supposed to make us look younger because this water types keep the skin hydrated. The reason is that the ionized water has various smaller clusters containing it.

This water type also has the benefit of aiding digestion since it helps to produce extra saliva which carries the food down to the digestive tract. You should also eat food with more fiber in it as the saliva works together with the fiber in the stomach to help get rid of toxic wastes from the body and enhance the metabolism. It is also supposed to be a good anti aging agent due to the effect of ionized water that has many antioxidants in it. The antioxidants are helping the body by getting rid of harmful free radicals that are basically a major cause of aging.

In addition it helps with weight loss since first of all drinking water regularly makes one eat less by curbing that constant hunger. Also the metabolism is effectively increased so that helps with burning the calories faster in the body. It is a great detoxificator since with drinking plenty of water, the toxins from the body get flushed out, especially when it comes to the kidneys. Sadly with age the kidneys are less equipped to do it on their own so they need outside help to perform their job the optimal way. This is where water comes into place.

Helps with minimizing the risk of various heart diseases such as heart attacks. Just by increasing the intake of fresh liquid, people are less prone to get heart attacks in their lives.

These are just some of the benefits of consuming fresh, pure and alkaline water. By picking up a glass and drinking more often you increase your health benefits and get to live longer as well.

Benefits Of Keeping The Brain Young With Physical Activities, Reading And Meditation

The human brain is an extremely complex organ. Despite rapid scientific progress, the knowledge about how the brain works in still evolving. The brain contains about 100 billion neurons, which are highly specialized nerve cells responsible for communicating information throughout the body. For each neuron, there are roughly anywhere from 1,000 to 10,000 synapses. A synapse is the connection between neurons that permits a neuron to pass an electrical or chemical signal to another neuron. Hormones and neurotransmitters are examples of chemical signals. The old adage of humans only using 10% of our brain is not true. Every part of the brain has a known function. Humans continue to make new neurons throughout life in response to mental activity. When you learn something new, your brain undergoes physical changes. The brain keeps growing in the frontal and temporal lobes well into middle-age, which can be associated with better emotional development and wisdom. The brain is, in fact, very much like a muscle which can be "bulked up" through exercise. Hence, it is possible to stimulate and challenge your brain as you get older to promote its continued growth. This means that the opposite also holds true drug use, poor nutrition, or other assaults on your brain can interfere with its development and health. This may be the explanation why Alzheimer's disease and other types of dementia cases are skyrocketing in the U.S. and many developed countries. So even if you haven't been leading the healthiest lifestyle thus far, making some positive changes now may still provide your brain what it needs to stay healthy as you age. The following are tips on how to keep your brain young and healthy.

Exercise

Research finds that with dementia, there is a shrinkage of the dendrites (branched projections of a neuron) that connect the neurons. There is also less production of neurotransmitters and the hippocampus gets smaller. Numerous studies found that aerobic exercise encourages your brain to work at optimum capacity by causing nerve cells to multiply, strengthening their interconnections, and protecting them from damage. For older people, aerobic exercise is very effective in boosting executive skills that includes planning, scheduling, multi-tasking, dealing with ambiguity and working memory (the ability to store short-term memory and process the information). So, if you want to boost your brain size, go for a brisk walk every day.

Challenge Your Mind

The brain is like a muscle. If you challenge it, it will get stronger. Mind-training activities stimulate blood flow, strengthen the synapses between neurons, and keep your brain fit as you age.

Reading challenging books

Learning a new language

Playing a musical instrument

Playing games such as crossword puzzles, Scrabble, and sudoku

Mastering a new hobby

Engaging in friendly debates

Meditation

As people age, their brain's lose weight and volume. These changes may start to occur in people as early as their mid to late 20s. Previous research has shown people who meditate to lose less brain mass over time than those who do not. In particular, research concluded people who meditated showed less of a decrease in their white brain matter. White brain matter acts as a connector and insulator for gray brain matter. It carries nerve impulses between the functional parts of the brain. Gray brain matter houses the various neurological centers of the brain, which direct speech, motor skills, memory, etc.

Meditation is something practiced by more than 15 million Americans and many more people around the world. It has its roots in eastern culture, but has been whole-heartedly embraced in western societies. It has a wide variety of benefits, including:

- Improves sleep

- Inner peace and tranquility

- Reduces chronic pain

- Reduces stress and anxiety

- Reduces depression

- Boosts attention

- Improves immunity

- Helps with weight loss

- Boosts memory

- Improves heart health and lowers blood pressure

- Improves wellbeing and allows for deeper relationships

Now it seems that meditation may also help to keep our brains young.

Interesting Experiments

A team of researchers from UCLA wondered if meditation preserves the gray matter of people who meditate as well. The researchers found meditation to have a widespread effect on the entire brain not just specific regions of the brain associated with meditation. The study compared people having years of meditation experience with those who had none. The meditators had an average of 20 years of experience with meditation practice. The age range of the of the study participants included people in their mid-20s to their late 70s. Nearly equal numbers of men and women participated in the study with 28 men and 22 women.

They found the meditators still experienced a decline in gray matter with age but less than non-meditators. The researchers noted the positive outcome of the study but caution people reviewing the results; they were unable to establish a direct link to meditation and the preservation of gray matter. Another UCLA study conducted in 2012, showed meditators to have more gyrification, folds in their brains, which may contribute to an ability process information faster than usual. Meditation appears to allow practitioners to maintain both white and gray matter and form increased connections in the brain; it seems to keep the brain young. Along with its positive effects on white and gray brain matter, meditation appears to have a positive effect on other body functions.

Anti-Aging Benefits Of Meditation

The youth preserving and renewing benefits of meditation include:

- Meditation increases DHEA, which facilitates the production of the hormones that maintain fat and mineral metabolism.

- An increase in Melatonin, which acts as antioxidant, supplies immune support and fights depression.

- A decrease in cortisol, the stress hormone that encourages the body to retain dangerous belly fat associated with heart disease and diabetes.

The Effects Of Meditation

Part of feeling and maintaining a youthful mental outlook centers around the quality of one's thinking patterns. Meditators learn to quiet mental chaos and build their ability to concentrate. They experience greater clarity of thought and tend to react less and respond more to circumstances. In short, they maintain their ability to be highly adaptive and think quickly with the additional benefit of choosing their response to situations rather than reacting to them.

How to Meditate

Meditators typically meditate at least twice a day for twenty minutes per sitting. Most schools of thought recommend meditation to start the day and to close it. However, a person may meditate whenever they have time in their schedule to accommodate it. Meditation is not an all or nothing proposition. It is also beneficial to meditate in shorter increments of time, sitting for 5, 10, or 15 minutes. There are also several different methods of meditation, including:

- Primordial Sound Meditation

- Mindfulness-Based Stress Reduction Zen

- Yoga Meditation (Kundalini)

- Focused Attention Meditation

- Open Monitoring Meditation

- Vipassana Meditation

- Loving Kindness Meditation (Metta Meditation)

- Mantra Meditation (OM Meditation)

- Qigong (Chi kung)

Getting Started

A person new to meditation needs to be patient; it takes time to train the mind to focus and settle into a meditation practice. The first step is to decide which from of meditation you wish to practice, and then learn how to do it. If possible, obtain the services of an expert, and there are also many books, DVD's and free information available online that can teach the exact steps of the particular method preferred. When beginning, try to meditate at the same time every day. If this is not possible, you can still meditate at different time.

Building a meditation practice is more important than when you do it. The benefits of a consistent meditation practice can develop in a few weeks with continued practice preserving your brain's youthful dynamics for years to come.

CONCLUSION

You are what you eat! you've certainly heard the expression many times, "You are what you eat." Have you ever really thought about what it means? And do you think about it when you're making food choices?

In some ways, we do become what we eat, literally. Have you ever seen an example of your blood plasma after eating a fast food hamburger? What was previously a clear liquid becomes cloudy with the fat and cholesterol that's absorbed from eating a high-fat hamburger.

And when you think about it, we also become what we don't eat. Our cholesterol can improve. When we're leaner and eating fewer animal products, then many other health and fitness issues are reduced. The incidence of Type II diabetes is reduced. Blood pressure falls into normal ranges. When you're healthier, you're taking fewer medications. Even if you have a prescription drug benefit in your health plan, you're still saving money with fewer co-payments on medications.

If you have a family history of high cholesterol or high blood pressure, then it's particularly

incumbent on you to revise your eating habits.

Life begins at the end of your comfort zone

Neale Donald Walsch

THE END!

Dear reader! I have a present for you! The first chapter of my new bestseller:

Quick Keto Reset Diet for Busy People

The Ultimate Keto Diet Book with Easy to Cook Ketogenic Diet Recipes for Weight Loss in 21 Days

By:

Nathalie Washington

Quick Keto Reset Diet for Busy People

The Ultimate Keto Diet Book with Easy to Cook Ketogenic Diet Recipes for Weight Loss in 21 Days

TABLE OF CONTENTS

INTRODUCTION

The Keto Diet has become quite a popular topic in the fitness community. It has been found to aid in the loss of weight and lowering the inflammation in the gut. New research has shown positive effects for both men and women adhering to a keto style diet.

Fluctuating hormones can cause pain, fatigue, and even depression. The link between hormones and cancer cannot be denied. A keto diet has shown to better regulate the endocrine system. By doing this, it decreases the incidence of some cancers, thyroid disease, and diabetes.

Slowly and carefully. A keotgenic diet should not be started at a full 100 percent. You should slowly decrease the amount of carbs you consume. Cutting the carbs too quickly can actually have a negative effect. It can stress the body and confuse it, thus causing a wild imbalance.

What is the Keto Diet?

First, a keto, or ketogenic diet, is designed to keep your body in more of a ketosis state. Ketosis is not abnormal. It is a state where your body is low on carbohydrate fuel. When this occurs, it starts to burn fat, rather than the carbs. The process produces ketones. The average person does not stay in a ketogenic state except during heavy exercise, such as CrossFit, or during pregnancy.

A ketogenic diet promotes very low carbohydrate and higher fat intake. The body will in turn, use fat to produce energy. This diet has also been shown to decrease autoimmune diseases, endocrine diseases, and also has cancer fighting properties.

Ketosis can be an issue with diabetics. This can occur if not using enough insulin.

A ketogenic diet helps to burn fat, thus losing weight. This low carb diet is similar to the Paleo Diet. We are a strong proponent of Paleo because it promotes higher protein for fuel instead of carbs. As we stated earlier, the keto diet uses fat rather than protein for fuel. A keto and paleo diet both burn fat while maintaining muscle.

Benefits Of Keto Diet

Here are some benefits of Keto Diet

Ketosis May Help Treat Cancer

Early research suggests that the keto diet may slow the growth of cancerous tumors. "Cancer cells have plenty of insulin receptors on them, making them flourish in environments high in blood sugar and insulin," says Brandon Olin, host of The Deskbound Podcast, which focuses on overcoming the damage of a sedentary lifestyle. "It's essentially giving cancer cells a source of fuel to feed on and grow." The research suggests ketone bodies may provide energy for your body without feeding the tumors.

Anxiety And Depression Diminish

While these findings are preliminary, in one study of mice, the keto diet helped reduce anxiety. The research suggests this could be due to the protective brain benefits of intake of healthy fats and low levels of sugar. A follow-up study found that mice exposed to a ketogenic diet while in utero showed less susceptibility to anxiety and depression than mice born to mothers who were not on the keto diet.

You'll Sleep Sounder

Many people on a ketogenic diet report sleeping much deeper, says Pamela Ellgen, a personal trainer and author of Sheet Pan Ketogenic. However, during the adjustment period (the first three to five days after you start keto), you may experience insomnia or difficulty staying asleep. This will end once your body adjusts to ketosis and burning stored fat. Then, you may find you're able to sleep longer, sleep deeper, and feel more relaxed and rested when you wake up.

Stronger Mental Performance

Mental clarity, an increased ability to focus and a better memory are other commonly reported benefits of eating a ketogenic diet.

Increasing intake of healthy fats with omega-3, such as those found in oily fish like salmon, tuna and mackerel, can improve mood and learning ability. This is because omega-3 increases a fatty acid called DHA that makes up between 15 to 30 per cent of our brain.

Keto Diet Recipes

Day 1

Breakfast

Keto Chicken Parmesan

Prep Time: 20 m
Cook Time: 8 m
Total Time: 28
2 servings

Ingredients

- 1 (8 ounce) skinless, boneless chicken breast
- 1 egg
- 1 tablespoon heavy whipping cream
- 1 1/2 ounces pork rinds, crushed
- 1 ounce grated Parmesan cheese

- 1/2 teaspoon salt
- 1/2 teaspoon garlic powder
- 1/2 teaspoon red pepper flakes (optional)
- 1/2 teaspoon ground black pepper
- 1/2 teaspoon Italian seasoning
- 1/2 cup jarred tomato sauce (such as Rao's®)
- 1/4 cup shredded mozzarella cheese
- 1 tablespoon ghee (clarified butter)

Instructions

- Set oven rack about 6 inches from the heat source and preheat the oven's broiler.
- Slice chicken breast through the middle horizontally from one side to within 1/2 inch of the other side. Open the two sides and spread them out like an open book. Pound chicken flat until about 1/2-inch thick.
- Beat egg and cream together in a bowl.
- Combine crushed pork rinds, Parmesan cheese, salt, garlic powder, red pepper flakes, ground black pepper, and Italian seasoning in bowl; transfer breading to a plate.
- Dip chicken into egg mixture; coat completely. Press chicken into breading; thickly coat both sides.
- Heat a skillet over medium-high heat; add ghee. Place chicken in the pan; cook until no longer pink in the center and the juices run clear, about 3 minutes per side. An instant-read thermometer inserted into the center should read at least 165 degrees F (74 degrees C). Be careful to keep breading in place.

- Transfer chicken to a baking sheet. Cover with tomato sauce; top with mozzarella cheese.
- Broil until cheese is bubbling and barely browned, about 2 minutes.

Nutrition Info

Calories: 442 cals

Lunch

Keto Chicken Enchilada Bowl

This Keto Chicken Enchilada Bowl is a low carb twist on a Mexican favorite!

Prep Time: 20 minutes
Cook Time: 30 minutes
Total Time: 50 minutes
Serving: 4

Ingredients

- 2 tablespoons coconut oil (for searing chicken)
- 1 pound of boneless, skinless chicken thighs
- 3/4 cup red enchilada sauce (recipe from Low Carb Maven)
- 1/4 cup water
- 1/4 cup chopped onion
- 4 oz can diced green chiles

Toppings (feel free to customize)

- 1 whole avocado, diced
- 1 cup shredded cheese (I used mild cheddar)
- 1/4 cup chopped pickled jalapenos
- 1/2 cup sour cream
- 1 roma tomato, chopped

Optional: serve over plain cauliflower rice (or mexican cauliflower rice) for a more complete meal!

Instructions

- In a pot or dutch oven over medium heat melt the coconut oil. Once hot, sear chicken thighs until lightly brown.

- Pour in enchilada sauce and water then add onion and green chiles. Reduce heat to a simmer and cover. Cook chicken for

17-25 minutes or until chicken is tender and fully cooked through to at least 165 degrees internal temperature.

- Careully remove the chicken and place onto a work surface. Chop or shred chicken (your preference) then add it back into the pot. Let the chicken simmer uncovered for an additional 10 minutes to absorb flavor and allow the sauce to reduce a little.

- To Serve, top with avocado, cheese, jalapeno, sour cream, tomato, and any other desired toppings. Feel free to customize these to your preference. Serve alone or over cauliflower rice if desired just be sure to update your personal nutrition info as needed.

Nutrition Info

Calories: 568 Calories
Total Carbs: 10.41g
Fiber: 4.27g
Net Carbs: 6.14g

Dinner

Keto Instant Pot Crack Chicken Recipe

Prep time: 5 mins
Cook time: 20 mins
Total time: 25 mins
Serves: 8 servings

Ingredients

- 2 slices bacon, chopped
- 2 lbs (910 g) boneless, skinless chicken breasts
- 2 (8 oz/227 g) blocks cream cheese
- ½ cup (120 ml) water
- 2 tablespoons apple cider vinegar
- 1 tablespoon dried chives
- 1½ teaspoons garlic powder
- 1½ teaspoons onion powder
- 1 teaspoon crushed red pepper flakes
- 1 teaspoon dried dill
- ¼ teaspoon salt
- ¼ teaspoon black pepper
- ½ cup (2 oz/57 g) shredded cheddar
- 1 scallion, green and white parts, thinly sliced

Instructions

Turn pressure cooker on, press "Sauté", and wait 2 minutes for the pot to heat up. Add the chopped bacon and cook until crispy. Transfer to a plate and set aside. Press "Cancel" to stop sautéing.

Add the chicken, cream cheese, water, vinegar, chives, garlic powder, onion powder, crushed red pepper flakes, dill, salt, and black pepper to the pot. Turn the pot on Manual, High Pressure for 15 minutes and then do a quick release.

Use tongs to transfer the chicken to a large plate, shred it with 2 forks, and return it back to the pot.

Stir in the cheddar cheese.

Top with the crispy bacon and scallion, and serve.

Nutrition Info

Calories: 437 Fat: 27.6 Potassium: 390 Net Carbs: 4.3 Carbohydrates: 4.5 Sodium: 420 Fiber: .2 Protein: 41.2

Day 2

Breakfast

Keto mushroom omelet

Looking for a quick and easy way to start your day? This hearty omelet is super healthy, and just takes a few minutes to make! Fresh mushrooms make a delicious filling. Enjoy this keto meal anytime

Time: 5 + 10 m

Ingredients

3 eggs
1 oz. butter, for frying
1 oz. shredded cheese
1/5 yellow onion
3 mushrooms
salt and pepper

Instructions

Crack the eggs into a mixing bowl with a pinch of salt and pepper. Whisk the eggs with a fork until smooth and frothy.

Add salt and spices to taste.

Melt butter in a frying pan. Once the butter has melted, pour in the egg mixture.

When the omelet begins to cook and get firm, but still has a little raw egg on top, sprinkle cheese, mushrooms and onion on top (optional).

Using a spatula, carefully ease around the edges of the omelet, and then fold it over in half. When it starts to turn golden brown underneath, remove the pan from the heat and slide the omelet on to a plate.

Tip!

Serve the omelet with a crispy, green salad with vinaigrette dressing on the side. Yum!

Nutrition Info

Calories: 510kcal

Lunch

Almond Coconut Curry on Veges

Total Time 15 minutes

Servings 4

Ingredients

For the curry mixture
For the veges

1 tsp coconut oil
400 ml coconut milk
2 cups mushrooms
125 g almond butter (100% ground almonds)
4 cups spinach
1 tbsp tomato paste
2 cups brocolli (chopped into florets)
1 tbsp curry powder

Instructions

For the curry mixture

- Put the coconut drain, almond spread, tomato glue and curry powder in a blender. Mix for around 20 seconds or until smooth.
- Add the curry blend to a pan on low-medium warmth and warmth for 10-15 minutes or until warmed through. Blend habitually to abstain from staying.

For the veges

- Heat the coconut oil in a container on medium-high warmth and include the broccoli and mushrooms. Sear for around 3 minutes. Include the spinach and warmth for one more moment.
- Serve the veges in a bowl with the curry blend poured over the best.

Recipe Notes:

You can make the almond margarine by granulating almonds in a sustenance processor.

The curry blend isolates whenever left to sit in the refrigerator for some time, so make certain to mix it completely before utilizing on the off chance that you have put away it in the ice chest.

Nutrition Info

Calories: 438, Fats: 41g, Protein: 11g, Net Carbs: 9g

Dinner

Chili Dog Casserole Recipe

Prep Time 15 minutes
Cook Time 45 to 50 minutes
Servings: 8

Ingredients

- 8 all-beef hotdogs (sliced in half lengthwise)
- 1 pound ground beef (80% lean)

- 1 small red pepper (diced)
- 1 small yellow onion (diced)
- 2 cloves minced garlic
- 1 cup low carb tomato sauce
- 1 cup water
- 2 tablespoons tomato paste
- 1 teaspoon Worcestershire sauce
- 1 tablespoon chili powder
- 1 teaspoon ground cumin
- 1/2 teaspoon celery salt
- 1 cup shredded cheddar cheese
- salt and pepper

Instructions

- Preheat the oven to 400°F and lightly grease a 7x9-inch glass baking dish with cooking spray.
- Line the bottom of the baking dish with hotdogs then set aside.
- Combine the ground beef, peppers, onions, and garlic in a large skillet over medium-high heat.
- Cook until the beef is browned, breaking it up into chunks with a wooden spoon.
- Stir in the tomato sauce, water, tomato paste, Worcestershire sauce, and seasonings.
- Bring to a boil then reduce heat and simmer on medium-low for 30 minutes.
- Spoon the chili over the hotdogs and sprinkle with cheese.
- Bake for 15 to 20 minutes until the cheese is hot and bubbling.
- Rest for 10 minutes before serving.

Nutrition Info

365 Calories
27g of Fat
24.5g of Protein
4.5g of Net Carbs

Day 3

Breakfast

Keto Pancakes

Prep Time: 0 hours 5 mins
Total Time: 0 hours 15 mins
Servingss: 10

Ingredients

- 1/2 c. almond flour
- 4 oz. cream cheese, softened
- 4 large eggs
- 1 tsp. lemon zest
- Butter, for frying and serving

Instructions

- In a medium bowl, whisk together almond flour, cream cheese, eggs, and lemon zest until smooth.

- In a nonstick skillet over medium heat, melt 1 tablespoon butter. Pour in about 3 tablespoons batter and cook until golden, 2 minutes. Flip and cook 2 minutes more. Transfer to a plate and continue with the rest of the batter.
- Serve topped with butter.

Lunch

Sesame Salmon w. Baby Bok Choy & Mushrooms

Ingredients

Main Dish

- 4 each 4-6 oz. salmon fillet
- 2 each portobello mushroom caps (or 8 oz. baby bella mushrooms)
- 4 each baby bok choy
- 1 tbsp toasted sesame seeds
- 1 ea green onion

Marinade

- 1 tbsp olive oil
- 1 tsp sesame oil
- 1 tbsp Coconut Aminos
- 1/2 inch Ginger grated (approx. 1 tsp.)
- 1/2 lemon juice
- 1/2 tsp Salt

- 1/2 tsp black pepper

Instructions

- Whisk together all of your marinade ingredients
- Drizzle half of the marinade on the salmon and turn to coat. Cover and refrigerate the salmon while it marinates for one hour.
- Preheat oven to 400.
- Prepare vegetables: Trim the rough ends from the bok choy and cut into halves. Slice the mushrooms into ½ inch pieces.
- Drizzle the remaining marinade over the vegetables and lay on a lined baking sheet.
- Place salmon, skin side down, on a lined baking sheet as well. Bake until salmon is cooked through, about 20 minutes.
- Top with sliced green onions and sesame seeds.

Dinner

Crab Stuffed Mushrooms With Cream Cheese

An easy recipe for crab stuffed mushrooms with cream cheese. Low carb, keto, and gluten free.

Prep Time 15 minutes
Cook Time 30 minutes
Servings 4 servings

Ingredients

- 20 ounces cremini (baby bella) mushrooms (20-25 individual mushrooms)
- 2 tablespoons finely grated parmesan cheese
- 1 tablespoon chopped fresh parsley
- salt

Filling:

- 4 ounces cream cheese softened to room temperature
- 4 ounces crab meat finely chopped
- 5 cloves garlic minced
- 1 teaspoon dried oregano
- 1/2 teaspoon paprika
- 1/2 teaspoon black pepper
- 1/4 teaspoon salt

Instructions

- Preheat the oven to 400 F. Prepare a baking sheet lined with parchment paper.
- Snap stems from mushrooms, discarding the stems and placing the mushroom caps on the baking sheet 1 inch apart from each other. Season the mushroom caps with salt.
- In a large mixing bowl, combine all filling ingredients and stir until well-mixed without any lumps of cream cheese. Stuff the mushroom caps with the mixture. Evenly sprinkle parmesan cheese on top of the stuffed mushrooms.

- Bake at 400 F until the mushrooms are very tender and the stuffing is nicely browned on top, about 30 minutes. Top with parsley and serve while hot.

Nutrition Info

Calories 160
Total Carb 5.5g 2%
Dietary Fiber 0.5g 1%
Sugars 0g
Protein 9g

Day 4

Breakfast

Jalapeño Popper Egg Cups

Prep Time: 0 hours 15 mins
Total Time: 0 hours 35 mins
Servingss: 4 - 6

Ingredients

- 12 slices bacon
- 10 large eggs
- 1/4 c. sour cream
- 1/2 c. shredded Cheddar
- 1/2 c. shredded mozzarella
- 2 jalapeños, 1 minced and 1 thinly sliced

- 1 tsp. garlic powder
- kosher salt
- Freshly ground black pepper
- nonstick cooking spray

Instructions

- Preheat oven to 375°.

- In a large skillet over medium heat, cook bacon until slightly browned but still pliable. Set aside on a paper towel-lined plate to drain.

- In a large bowl, whisk together eggs, sour cream, cheeses, minced jalapeño and garlic powder. Season with salt and pepper.

- Using nonstick cooking spray, grease a muffin tin. Line each well with one slice of bacon, then pour egg mixture into each muffin cup until about two-thirds of the way to the top. Top each muffin with a jalapeño slice.

- Bake for 20 minutes, or until the eggs no longer look wet. Cool slightly before removing from the muffin tin. Serve.

Nutrition Info

Calories: 230kcal

Lunch

Caprese Tuna Salad Stuffed Tomatoes

Prep Time: 10 minutes
Servings: Serves 1

Ingredients

- 1 medium tomato
- 1 (5oz) can tuna, very well drained
- 2 tsp balsamic vinegar
- 1 TBSP chopped mozzarella {1/4 oz.}
- 1 TBSP chopped fresh basil
- 1 TBSP chopped green onion

Instructions

- Cut the top 1/4-inch off the tomato. Use a spoon to scoop out the insides of the tomato. Set aside while you make the tuna salad.
- Stir together the drained tuna, balsamic vinegar, mozzarella, basil, and green onion. Put the tuna salad in the hollowed out tomato, and enjoy!
- Note: I prefer using fresh mozzarella but any mozzarella is good in here.

Nutrition Info

Calories per serving: 196
Fat per serving: 4.9g

Dinner

Lemon Butter Sauce for Fish

Prep: 5 mins
Cook: 10 mins
Total: 15 mins
Servings: 2

Ingredients

Lemon Butter Sauce:

- 60 g / 4 tbsp unsalted butter , cut into pieces
- 1 tbsp fresh lemon juice
- Salt and finely ground pepper

Crispy Pan Fried Fish:

- 2 x thin white fish fillets (120-150g / 4-5oz each), skinless boneless (I used Bream, Note 1)
- Salt and pepper
- 2 tbsp white flour
- 2 tbsp oil (I use canola)

Serving:

- Lemon wedges

- Finely chopped parsley, optional

Instructions

- Place the butter in a light coloured saucepan or small skillet over medium heat.

  - Melt butter then leave on the stove, whisking / stirring very now and then. When the butter turns golden brown and it smells nutty - about 3 minutes, remove from stove immediately and pour into small bowl.
- Add lemon juice and a pinch of salt and pepper. Stir then taste when it has cooled slightly. Adjust lemon/salt to taste.

- Set aside - it will stay pourable for 20 - 30 minutes. See Note 3 for storing.

Did you like the preview? You can buy the book on Amazon

Quick Keto Reset Diet for Busy People

The Ultimate Keto Diet Book with Easy to Cook Ketogenic Diet
Recipes for Weight Loss in 21 Days

By Nathalie Washington

I want to thank you for reading this book. I hope that you received value from it. If you received value from my book, leave a 5 stars review for this title.

THANK YOU!

NATHALIE WASHINGTON 2019